Introduction

The Struggle for Balance in Tech

Welcome to "Eat, Pray, Code: A Guide to Maintaining Work-Life Balance in the Tech Industry." If you've picked up this book, chances are you're either working in tech or aspire to be part of this fascinating yet demanding world. It's an industry that moves at the speed of light, fueled by constant innovation, tight deadlines, and ceaseless ambition. It's also a realm where the word "balance" often seems like a foreign concept.

The high-stress environment in the tech industry is almost legendary. Late nights, early mornings, and weekends spent in front of a screen aren't uncommon. While this can create a culture of productivity and groundbreaking developments, it also generates a vortex that can suck you in, making you lose sight of everything else that matters—your health, relationships, and overall well-being.

For many, the first thing that falls by the wayside is a balanced diet, hence the stereotype of a programmer living on pizza and energy drinks. Physical fitness often comes next, as the lure of solving a particularly challenging problem or meeting a tight deadline keeps us shackled to our desks. This sedentary lifestyle brings with it a host of health problems, ranging from the mild—like wrist and back pain—to more severe, like obesity and heart issues.

Then comes the toll on mental and emotional health. Stress, burnout, and isolation can become a part of the daily routine, affecting not only your work performance but also your relationships and your sense of self. The paradox here is that while the tech industry has given us tools to connect more easily than ever before, we are often ironically disconnected from our own selves and the people around us.

But it doesn't have to be this way.

This book is designed to be a comprehensive guide to reclaiming your life while succeeding in your tech career. In the following chapters, we will explore how to nourish your body and mind ("Eat"), cultivate mental and emotional well-being ("Pray"), and implement strategies to excel in your tech career without burning out ("Code").

So, who is this book for? It's for the software engineer who wants to be on top of his game without sacrificing his health. It's for the tech startup entrepreneur buried under the weight of both coding and running a business. It's for the data scientist, the system administrator, the product manager, and any other tech professional who wants to find a fulfilling work-life balance.

It's not just a book; it's your blueprint for a balanced, fulfilling life in tech.

Welcome to your journey toward eating well, nurturing your spirit, and coding your way to success. Let's begin.

Eat: Nourishing Your Body and Mind

Eating Right for Maximum Productivity

The Fuel Behind the Code

Food is fuel. Just as you wouldn't expect a car to run smoothly on poor-quality gas, you can't expect your brain—the powerhouse of your coding ability—to function at its peak on a diet of fast food, sugary snacks, and caffeine overloads. In the tech world, where the demand for cognitive function is extraordinarily high, what you eat can significantly impact your performance, focus, and productivity.

What Goes In Must Come Out—In Code!

Imagine a scenario where you have a tight deadline, and you've chosen to consume high-sugar, high-caffeine foods to keep you awake and alert. Initially, you may experience a surge of energy, often referred to as a 'sugar rush.' But once that fades, you're left feeling lethargic, distracted, and unable to focus—the dreaded 'sugar crash.'

Your brain relies on a steady supply of energy, and the spikes and crashes associated with a poor diet can make maintaining a consistent level of productivity almost impossible. It's not just about avoiding certain foods, though; it's about embracing a diet that nourishes both your body and your mind.

The Good Stuff: What Should You Eat?

Complex Carbohydrates: Whole grains, fruits, and vegetables provide slow-releasing energy that can help maintain your concentration levels throughout the day.

Proteins: Amino acids found in proteins are the building blocks of neurotransmitters, the brain's messengers. Lean meat, fish, dairy, and legumes are excellent sources of protein that can enhance cognitive function.

Healthy Fats: Omega-3 fatty acids found in foods like fish, flaxseeds, and walnuts are known to boost brain power. They can also help manage mood, which is especially helpful when dealing with the ups and downs of tech life.

Vitamins and Minerals: Leafy greens, fruits, and vegetables are loaded with vitamins like B, C, and K, which have been proven to improve memory, attention, and overall brain function.

Snacking Smart

Techies are known for their love of snacking, often because it's a way to sustain energy during long coding sessions. However, choosing the right snacks is crucial. Instead of reaching for a bag of chips or a can of soda, consider these alternatives:

Nuts and Seeds: A handful of almonds or pumpkin seeds can provide the quick protein and healthy fat fix you need.

Fresh Fruits: Sliced apples, bananas, or a cup of mixed berries can offer a natural sugar kick without the subsequent crash.

Yogurt and Granola: A small bowl can provide both protein and complex carbohydrates, sustaining you for a longer period.

A Note on Hydration

Dehydration can severely affect your cognitive abilities, including focus and memory. Make it a habit to drink water throughout the day, and if you're looking for a caffeine fix, consider healthier options like green tea, which also contains antioxidants.

Conclusion: The Balanced Plate, The Balanced Code

While the "Eat" in "Eat, Pray, Code" may appear to be the simplest part of the equation, it's one that should not be neglected. Remember, maintaining a well-rounded, nutritious diet isn't just beneficial for your physical health; it's crucial for your productivity and success in the tech industry. As the saying goes, "You are what you eat," and in the world of tech, you certainly want to be sharp, efficient, and at the top of your game.

The Science of Brain Foods

The Brain-Gut Connection

Most of us are familiar with the saying, "You are what you eat." What you may not know is that this old adage holds scientific truth, especially when it comes to brain function. The gut and the brain are more connected than we've ever imagined, thanks to the "gut-brain axis," a bidirectional communication system between the central nervous system and the gastrointestinal tract. Certain foods can actually boost neurotransmitters, reduce inflammation, and aid in the creation of brain cells, thereby affecting our cognitive abilities, mood, and overall mental well-being.

Nutritional Neuroscience: A Growing Field

Nutritional neuroscience is an emerging discipline dedicated to understanding how various components of food influence our brains. Studies in this field have revealed specific nutrients that can have a profound effect on our cognitive functions, emotional well-being, and even our professional performance—of particular interest for those in the tech industry.

The Mighty Omega-3s

Omega-3 fatty acids, particularly EPA and DHA, are among the most well-researched brain foods. They are essential for brain health, including cognitive function and mental well-being. Research has shown that individuals who consume a diet rich in Omega-3s perform better in cognitive tests and are less susceptible to conditions like depression and anxiety. Sources of Omega-3s include fatty fish (such as salmon, mackerel, and sardines), flaxseeds, and walnuts.

Antioxidants and Cognitive Function

Antioxidants like flavonoids, found in fruits like berries and grapes, have shown promise in improving cognitive functions like memory and attention. They do so by reducing oxidative stress and inflammation, which can impair brain functions over time. Adding a handful of berries to your morning oatmeal or as a snack can go a long way.

Protein and Neurotransmitters

Proteins are the building blocks of neurotransmitters, which are chemicals that transmit signals in the brain. Amino acids like tryptophan can help produce serotonin, often termed the "feel-good hormone," while tyrosine is crucial in the production of dopamine, which influences mood and pleasure. Foods rich in high-quality protein like lean meat, eggs, and legumes can thus contribute to a balanced mood and enhanced concentration.

Vitamins for the Brain

Certain vitamins, notably B vitamins like B6, B9 (folate), and B12, have been found to be essential for brain health. They aid in the formation of brain chemicals like dopamine and serotonin, which can enhance mood, and are involved in the maintenance of the brain's nerve sheaths. Lack of these vitamins has been linked to higher levels of fatigue and depression.

Applying the Science in Tech Life

Understanding the science of brain foods can be a game-changer in the tech industry, where cognitive prowess is often the key to success. Whether you're debugging code, brainstorming innovative solutions, or dealing with the stress of startup life, the foods you choose can make a real difference. Make it a point to incorporate these nutrient-rich foods into your daily diet and notice the improvements not just in your work but in your overall quality of life.

In our next section, we'll explore the importance of physical exercise in maintaining a balanced life in the tech world. Just like the right foods fuel your brain, the right exercises fuel your overall well-being, making you a more effective and happier tech professional.

Physical Exercise: Not Just for Athletes

The Missing Link

When we talk about nourishing the body and mind for maximum productivity in the tech industry, we often overlook a critical element: physical exercise. It's easy to dismiss physical activity as something reserved for athletes or fitness enthusiasts, but science tells a different story. Exercise isn't just about building muscles or losing weight; it's also about enhancing brain function, reducing stress, and improving overall well-being—all critical factors for anyone in the high-pressure tech world.

Mind-Body Connection: It's Real

The connection between physical activity and mental acuity is well-documented. Exercise has been shown to improve cognitive functions like memory, attention, and problem-solving. It increases blood flow to the brain, enriching it with oxygen and essential nutrients. Physical exercise also stimulates the release of hormones like endorphins and serotonin, which can boost mood and reduce feelings of stress and anxiety.

Exercise and Creativity

For tech professionals who often need to think outside the box—whether it's solving a tricky programming issue or conceptualizing a new product—exercise can be a creativity catalyst. Physical activity can help "unstick" mental blocks and facilitate creative thinking. You might find that the solution to a problem you've been struggling with suddenly becomes clear during or after some form of physical exercise.

What Kind of Exercise Works Best?

You don't need to become a marathon runner or a gym rat to experience the benefits of physical activity. The key is to find something you enjoy and can incorporate into your routine. Here are some options:

- Cardio Workouts: Activities like jogging, cycling, and swimming are excellent for enhancing cardiovascular health and boosting endurance, which can indirectly improve mental stamina.
- Strength Training: Lifting weights or using resistance bands can improve muscle tone and strength, which can translate into better stamina for long coding sessions.
- Mind-Body Practices: Yoga, tai chi, and Pilates are not just good for your body but also have mindfulness elements that can help improve focus and reduce stress.
- Quick Office Exercises: If you're pressed for time, even simple exercises like jumping jacks, push-ups, or stretches done for 10 minutes can make a difference.

A Tech-Friendly Exercise Routine

To make it easier for tech professionals to incorporate exercise into their busy schedules, consider setting aside specific "exercise blocks" during your week. Use reminders or apps to prompt you and try pairing exercise with other activities. For instance, you could take walking meetings or do some quick stretches while your code is compiling.

Conclusion: A Synergistic Approach

In the tech industry, where cognitive function and mental well-being are critical, adopting a holistic approach that includes proper nutrition and regular physical exercise is not a luxury; it's a necessity. So, the next time you reach for a snack to fuel your coding session or take a break to clear your mind, consider pairing it with some form of physical activity. Your body, your brain, and your code will thank you.

Stay tuned for the next chapter, where we delve into the "Pray" part of "Eat, Pray, Code," focusing on mental and emotional well-being in the tech world. Because nourishing your body and mind is just the beginning—sustaining it requires a balanced soul.

Pray: Mental and Emotional Well-being

The Importance of Mindfulness

Unplugging to Recharge

The "Pray" in "Eat, Pray, Code" isn't strictly about religious or spiritual practice—although it can be, if that's what resonates with you. In the context of this book, "Pray" serves as a metaphor for the deliberate, focused time and energy we should devote to our inner selves. One of the most effective ways to do this is through the practice of mindfulness.

What Is Mindfulness?

Mindfulness is the mental state achieved by focusing your awareness on the present moment while calmly acknowledging and accepting your feelings, thoughts, and bodily sensations. In an industry like tech, where multitasking and constant problem-solving are the norms, mindfulness can provide the space and clarity we need to function at our best—emotionally, mentally, and professionally.

The Scientific Backing

Multiple studies have shown that mindfulness can help reduce stress, improve attention, and enhance emotional regulation—essential skills for anyone working in a high-pressure tech environment. The practice has also been associated with physiological benefits, such as lower blood pressure and improved immune response, which can be particularly beneficial when you're balancing long hours and tight deadlines.

Mindfulness and Emotional Intelligence

Being mindful also improves your emotional intelligence, a skill increasingly recognized as vital in the professional world. Emotional intelligence enables you to navigate complex social interactions, manage stress, and make better decisions—critical abilities in team-oriented tech settings.

Simple Mindfulness Practices for Techies

You don't have to meditate for an hour each day to experience the benefits of mindfulness (though that would certainly be great). Here are some quick and easy ways to incorporate mindfulness into your daily routine:

- Deep Breathing: Take a few minutes each day to breathe deeply and consciously. This simple act can help lower stress hormones and calm your mind.
- Mindful Eating: Instead of eating in front of your computer, try focusing solely on your meal. Notice the textures, flavors, and smells. This will not only enhance your eating experience but also give your brain a much-needed break.
- The Five-Minute Walk: Step away from your workspace and go for a brief walk. Use this time to focus on your senses. What do you see, hear, feel? This short break can reset your brain and improve focus.
- Single-Tasking: Choose a specific task and dedicate your full attention to it, avoiding the temptation to multi-task. You'll probably find that you complete the task more efficiently and effectively.

Integrating Mindfulness into Your Workday

Consider setting aside specific times for these practices or integrate them into your existing routines. You might start your day with a deep-breathing exercise, practice mindful eating during lunch, and take a five-minute walk in the afternoon when your energy starts to dip.

Conclusion: A Mindful Tech Life

The demands of the tech industry aren't going to change. There will always be another problem to solve, another code to debug, another project to manage. But by incorporating mindfulness into your daily routine, you're not just surviving these challenges—you're thriving amidst them. It makes the "Pray" in "Eat, Pray, Code" not an optional add-on but an essential component of a balanced, fulfilling life in tech.

Next, we'll dive into the "Code" part of "Eat, Pray, Code," where we'll discuss practical strategies for maintaining a balanced approach to your professional tasks and responsibilities. Stay tuned!

Meditation and Stress Relief

Stress: The Silent Productivity Killer

In the fast-paced world of technology, stress often comes with the territory. High expectations, tight deadlines, and an ever-changing landscape can make the tech industry an exciting but stressful place to work. Stress, if left unchecked, can wreak havoc on your mental and physical health, impairing your ability to solve problems and think creatively—skills that are crucial in this field. That's where meditation comes in.

What is Meditation?

Meditation is a mental exercise that involves relaxation, focus, and awareness. It is not so much a way to "think" but a way to "un-think"—to clear your mind, even for just a few minutes, to regain balance and inner peace. Various forms of meditation exist, from mindfulness meditation to transcendental meditation, but all aim to achieve a calmer state of mind.

The Science Behind Meditation and Stress Relief

Studies have shown that regular meditation can dramatically reduce the stress hormone cortisol, improve focus, increase cognitive flexibility, and even boost emotional well-being. Neuroscientists have found that meditation can change the structure and function of the brain in ways that promote mental health, such as increasing the density of gray matter in regions linked to memory and stress regulation.

How Meditation Fits into the Tech World

One might assume that meditation and tech are worlds apart—one involves unplugging and looking inward, while the other focuses on coding, hardware, and endless lines of logic. However, the two can be deeply interconnected.

Meditation can serve as a tool for mental debugging—a way to clear the mind and enhance cognitive abilities. In an industry where sharp thinking and problem-solving are key, meditation can be your secret weapon. Top tech companies like Google even offer mindfulness and meditation programs, recognizing the value of mental well-being in the workplace.

Simple Meditation Techniques for Beginners

Getting started with meditation doesn't require special equipment or a large time commitment. Here are some easy ways to begin:

- Breath Awareness: Sit comfortably and focus solely on your breath. Inhale and exhale naturally, concentrating on the sensation of the air moving in and out of your nostrils or your belly rising and falling.
- Body Scan: Lie down or sit comfortably. Starting from the top of your head, slowly scan down through your body, being aware of any tension or discomfort.
- Mindful Walking: Take a walk at a natural pace. Pay attention to how your body moves and how it feels to touch the ground.
- Guided Meditation: Use an app or video to guide you through a meditation session. This can be particularly useful for beginners who find it difficult to focus.

Integrating Meditation into Your Daily Routine

You don't have to meditate for hours to experience its benefits. Even just 5-10 minutes a day can make a significant difference. You could take a meditation break instead of a coffee break, meditate during your commute, or dedicate a few minutes before bed to unwind.

Conclusion: From Stressed to Centered

The "Pray" aspect in "Eat, Pray, Code" reflects more than just a call for spiritual or religious observance; it represents the mental and emotional nourishment that comes from practices like meditation. In the high-stress atmosphere of the tech industry, carving out time for meditation isn't just good for your peace of mind—it's essential for sustained productivity and creativity.

The Role of Spirituality

Beyond Code: The Spiritual Dimension

The "Pray" in "Eat, Pray, Code" signifies more than mindfulness and meditation; it also invites us to explore the realm of spirituality. Whether you identify with a particular faith, hold personal beliefs, or are just open to greater existential questions, spirituality can offer a meaningful way to cope with stress, find purpose, and attain a deeper sense of satisfaction in your tech career and life in general.

What Is Spirituality?

Spirituality is a broad concept, often described as the connection to something greater than oneself, which can involve a search for meaning in life. It is often linked to religion, but the two are not synonymous. Spirituality can encompass personal growth, a concern for peace and social justice, or a deep appreciation for the arts and nature.

Spirituality and Emotional Resilience

The tech industry is full of ups and downs. Projects get canceled, code breaks, and deadlines sometimes seem impossible. During these turbulent times, spirituality can act as an emotional anchor, providing the resilience needed to weather the storms of disappointment, stress, and failure. Spiritual practices can help you develop virtues like patience, humility, and perseverance—qualities that can be particularly useful in your professional journey.

Spiritual Practices for a Balanced Life

Spiritual practices can take many shapes and forms. Here are some you might consider integrating into your routine:

- Prayer or Reflection: Taking a few moments each day for prayer or reflective thinking can provide you with valuable insights and a sense of peace.
- Gratitude Journal: Keeping a gratitude journal can shift your focus from what's lacking or stressful to what's abundant and positive in your life.
- Community Involvement: Engaging in community service can be a deeply spiritual experience, fostering a sense of connection and shared humanity.
- Mindful Connection with Nature: Spend some time outdoors, paying full attention to the natural world around you. This can be a form of spiritual renewal.
- Reading Spiritual Texts: This could be scripture, poetry, or philosophical texts—anything that resonates with you and offers guidance or inspiration.

Integrating Spirituality into Your Work Life

Balancing a spiritual practice with a demanding tech career may seem challenging but it's far from impossible. Small changes can make a big difference:

You could start your day with a brief meditation or prayer session.

Take 'spiritual breaks' to read something uplifting or simply step outside to appreciate nature.

Practice mindful communication, bringing qualities of empathy and active listening to your workplace interactions.

Conclusion: Spirituality as a Source of Strength

In an industry that thrives on logic and rationality, the benefits of spirituality might seem counterintuitive or even irrelevant. However, as we've discussed, it can offer emotional resilience, foster community, and provide a sense of greater purpose—advantages that are as practical as they are profound.

So, the next time you're facing a complex coding problem or are stressed about meeting a deadline, remember that you have tools that go beyond your technical skills and intellectual capabilities. The "Pray" in "Eat, Pray, Code" is an invitation to tap into these deeper resources, rounding out a holistic approach to life and work in the tech industry.

In the next section, we'll move to the "Code" component of "Eat, Pray, Code," where we'll look at achieving excellence without burning out. Stay tuned!

Building Emotional Resilience

Facing the Inevitable Ups and Downs

In the tech world, volatility is a given. Whether it's the thrill of solving a complex problem, the high of launching a new product, or the stress that comes with unexpected glitches and tight deadlines, emotional highs and lows are part of the package. This roller-coaster ride can be exhilarating but also exhausting. That's why building emotional resilience is crucial for long-term success and well-being in this demanding field.

What Is Emotional Resilience?

Emotional resilience is the ability to adapt to stressful situations and to recover more quickly from setbacks. It's not about avoiding stress—something almost impossible to do in tech—but about managing and learning from it. Resilience equips you with the mental and emotional tools to navigate challenges, ensuring that stress and failure don't derail you but rather contribute to your growth.

The Importance of Emotional Resilience in Tech

In an industry where disruption is the norm, being emotionally resilient can make the difference between a long, fulfilling career and one that leaves you burned out and disillusioned. Resilient individuals are better able to cope with the demands of a fast-paced environment, handle pressure without crumbling, and adapt to change more readily.

Strategies for Building Emotional Resilience

Here are some effective ways to build your emotional resilience:

- Mindfulness Practices: As we've discussed earlier, mindfulness can help you become more aware of your emotional state, making it easier to regulate your reactions.
- Support Networks: Don't underestimate the power of a strong support network. Friends, family, and even professional connections can offer emotional support, practical advice, and a different perspective.
- Positive Framing: Learn to reframe challenges as opportunities for growth. This isn't about ignoring problems but about approaching them from a more empowered standpoint.
- Coping Skills: Develop a toolbox of coping mechanisms, such as deep breathing, exercise, or even a favorite inspirational quote, to turn to in stressful moments.
- Setting Boundaries: In a field that often glorifies overwork, setting clear work-life boundaries is a form of emotional self-care. Know when to step back and recharge.

Small Steps for Big Gains

You don't have to overhaul your life overnight to become more emotionally resilient. Small, consistent actions can yield significant results. Start by identifying one or two strategies that resonate with you and integrate them into your daily routine. As you become more adept at managing stress and bouncing back from setbacks, you'll find that these practices have a cumulative effect, equipping you with the emotional strength to face whatever challenges your tech career throws at you.

Conclusion: The "Pray" in Resilience

Emotional resilience forms a vital part of the "Pray" component in "Eat, Pray, Code." It's about investing in your inner strength so that you can meet external challenges more effectively. As you cultivate emotional resilience, you don't just improve your capacity to cope with stress and setbacks; you enhance your ability to find joy, meaning, and satisfaction in your work and life.

Up next, we'll delve into the "Code" section of "Eat, Pray, Code," focusing on sustainable practices that will help you excel in your tech career without burning out. Stay tuned!

Code: Succeeding without Burning Out

Agile Life Management

The Relentless Push for Excellence

In the world of tech, the pace is often set to "sprint." There's a constant drive to optimize, innovate, and disrupt. It's a world of late nights and early mornings, of pushing the envelope and redefining what's possible. But in this relentless pursuit of excellence, it's all too easy to burn out. That's where the concept of Agile Life Management comes in.

What is Agile Life Management?

You're probably familiar with Agile as a project management framework commonly used in software development. It emphasizes flexibility, collaboration, and adaptability. Agile Life Management applies these principles to managing your life, especially your work-life balance. It's about becoming the 'Product Owner' of your life, prioritizing tasks effectively, and iterating your way to a balanced, fulfilling existence.

Why Agile?

Agile methodologies prioritize "individuals and interactions over processes and tools." This means that you, your well-being, and your interactions with others take precedence over rigid life structures. Adopting an Agile mindset allows you to adapt to changes more efficiently, whether their project requirements at work or unexpected life events.

Implementing Agile Principles in Life

Here's how to adapt Agile principles to manage your life more efficiently and avoid burnout:

- Sprints: Divide your life's tasks and goals into short, manageable sprints. Each sprint could last a week or a month, during which you focus on completing a set of prioritized tasks.
- Stand-ups: Start your day with a quick mental 'stand-up' to review what you've done, what you plan to do, and any obstacles in your way. This keeps you focused and allows you to adapt your plans as needed.
- Retrospectives: At the end of each sprint, take time to review what worked, what didn't, and what could be improved. Use this reflection to plan your next sprint better.
- Backlog Management: Keep a 'backlog' of tasks, dreams, and goals. Regularly review and prioritize this list, adding items to your upcoming sprints as appropriate.
- Iteration: Life is unpredictable. Using an Agile approach means you can pivot and adapt, iterating on your life plans as circumstances change.

The Balance between 'Eat,' 'Pray,' and 'Code'

Agile Life Management isn't just about optimizing your work tasks; it's about achieving a balanced portfolio of life activities. This balance is what "Eat, Pray, Code" strives for. You 'sprint' not just through your coding tasks but also through your wellness activities ('Eat') and your mental and emotional well-being practices ('Pray').

Avoiding Burnout through Agile Life Management

The biggest advantage of applying Agile methodologies to your life could be the prevention of burnout. By continually reassessing your priorities and adapting to change, you can allocate time for relaxation, renewal, and skill development. You learn to work smarter, not harder, thereby preserving your mental and emotional well-being.

Conclusion: Code with Agility, Live with Agility

The "Code" in "Eat, Pray, Code" is about more than just writing software or building digital solutions. It's about applying the same focus, adaptability, and excellence to every aspect of your life. By using Agile Life Management, you ensure that you're not just succeeding in your tech career but also building a life that's robust, balanced, and fulfilling.

In the coming sections, we'll delve deeper into other strategies and tools that can help you navigate the complexities of a tech career while keeping your well-being front and center. Stay tuned!

The 80/20 Principle in Coding

The Perpetual Race Against Time

In the tech industry, the clock never seems to stop. There's always another feature to build, another bug to fix, another deadline looming on the horizon. This constant pressure can make coding a source of stress rather than a fulfilling creative process. But what if you could achieve more by actually doing less? Enter the 80/20 Principle, a concept that can revolutionize how you approach coding—and life.

What is the 80/20 Principle?

The 80/20 Principle, also known as the Pareto Principle, states that roughly 80% of effects come from 20% of causes. In the context of coding, this means that a significant portion of your productivity, efficiency, or impact can often be attributed to a small set of tasks, skills, or even lines of code. Understanding this principle can dramatically shift how you allocate your time and energy.

How the 80/20 Principle Applies to Coding

Here are some areas where the 80/20 principle can be effectively applied in the coding world:

- Debugging: Often, 80% of bugs come from 20% of the code. Focus on identifying and refining this problematic segment.
- Feature Development: Not all features are created equal. Some will be used frequently by many users, while others may rarely see the light of day. Prioritize building and refining the features that will make the most significant impact.

- Skill Mastery: In any programming language, understanding a core 20% of the language's capabilities can allow you to accomplish about 80% of what you need to do.
- Code Review: Instead of getting lost in the weeds, focus your code reviews on the most crucial 20% of the changes—those that have the most significant implications for performance, security, or maintainability.

Practical Steps for Applying the 80/20 Principle

Identify the Core 20%: Whether it's tasks for the week, coding challenges, or team responsibilities, identify the critical 20% that will yield the most significant results.

- Prioritize: Once you've identified the core 20%, make these your highest priority. Schedule them during your peak productivity hours.
- Eliminate or Delegate: What about the less impactful 80%? Evaluate whether these tasks are necessary. Can they be eliminated, automated, or delegated?
- Iterate: The 80/20 Principle isn't a one-time exercise. Regularly review your tasks, projects, and even your career trajectory to identify new "core 20%" areas.

Balancing the 80/20 Rule with 'Eat' and 'Pray'

In the larger context of "Eat, Pray, Code," the 80/20 Principle serves as a tool for balance. By focusing your coding efforts on the most impactful tasks, you free up time for nourishing your body ('Eat') and maintaining mental and emotional well-being ('Pray').

Conclusion: Achieve More by Focusing on Less

The 80/20 Principle challenges the notion that more hours spent coding equals more productivity. By honing in on the most critical tasks, you can not only be more productive but also achieve a better work-life balance, effectively embodying the spirit of "Eat, Pray, Code."

In the next section, we'll explore how to keep evolving in your tech career without sacrificing your health or happiness.

Avoiding Burnout

The Fine Line Between Passion and Exhaustion

The tech industry is built on passion—passion for innovation, for solving complex problems, and for making an impact. Yet, there's a thin line between passion and burnout, especially in a sector where the next big thing is always just around the corner. The term 'burnout' isn't just a buzzword; it's a real and pervasive issue that can deeply affect your health, happiness, and career longevity.

Defining Burnout

Burnout is a state of emotional, physical, and mental exhaustion, often resulting from prolonged stress or overwork. It manifests through symptoms like decreased productivity, disengagement, physical illness, and emotional volatility. In an industry that often operates in 'sprints,' the toll on individuals can be high.

Recognizing the Early Signs

Before diving into how to avoid burnout, it's essential to recognize its early indicators. This can range from mild symptoms like feeling tired often or finding it hard to focus, to more significant signs like dread for work, reduced job performance, and social withdrawal. Awareness is the first step towards prevention.

Strategies for Avoiding Burnout

Here are some strategies that can help you dodge the burnout bullet:

- Set Boundaries: Create clear distinctions between work and personal time. This could mean setting 'office hours' at home if you're remote, or consciously 'switching off' after a certain time.

- Take Breaks: Even short breaks, like a walk around the block or a few minutes of deep breathing, can do wonders for your mental state.
- Learn to Say No: It's tempting to take on every challenge that comes your way, but overcommitting will only set you up for failure and stress.
- Prioritize Self-Care: Exercise, eat balanced meals, get enough sleep—these aren't luxuries; they are necessities for long-term career success.
- Seek Support: Don't underestimate the power of a support network. Speak openly about your experiences with trusted colleagues, friends, or mentors who can provide emotional support and possibly even practical solutions.

Integrating 'Eat,' 'Pray,' and 'Code' for a Balanced Life

In the larger framework of "Eat, Pray, Code," avoiding burnout is integral to maintaining the balance that we strive for. While you focus on your coding goals ('Code'), do not neglect the importance of nourishing your body ('Eat') and investing in your mental and emotional well-being ('Pray'). All three aspects need to be in harmony for you to thrive in the tech industry without the shadow of burnout looming over you.

Conclusion: A Sustainable Path Forward

Avoiding burnout isn't just about self-preservation; it's about setting yourself up for a fulfilling, sustainable career in tech. By taking proactive steps to maintain a work-life balance and listening to your body and mind's signals, you can continue to push the boundaries of what's possible in tech without pushing yourself to the brink of burnout.

In our final section, we'll summarize the key points from each part of "Eat, Pray, Code" and offer a roadmap for how to implement these principles in your daily life.

Finding Your Coding 'Zen'

The Myth of the '10x Engineer'

In the tech world, there's a widely circulated myth about the '10x Engineer'—the individual who is purportedly ten times more productive than the average coder. While this concept can motivate some, it can also serve as a dangerous trap, pushing people towards unattainable expectations and inevitable burnout. But what if there was a different way to approach coding, one that centers on achieving a state of 'Zen'—a balanced, focused, and harmonious work state?

What is Coding 'Zen'?

Finding your Coding 'Zen' means discovering a sense of balance, focus, and flow in your work. It's a mental state where you are fully engaged in coding, not just as a task but as a fulfilling activity that brings you joy, challenges your skills, and offers a sense of accomplishment. It's about being in 'the zone,' where the code seems to write itself and solutions appear almost organically.

Why Strive for Coding 'Zen'?

Achieving a state of Coding 'Zen' brings several benefits:

- Improved Focus: Your mind is sharp, allowing you to solve complex problems more efficiently.
- Reduced Stress: The work is engaging but not stressful, balancing your mental load.
- Enhanced Creativity: You are more likely to come up with innovative solutions and approaches.
- Increased Satisfaction: Achieving a state of flow in your work leads to greater job satisfaction.

How to Find Your Coding 'Zen'

Here are some techniques to help you reach this state:

- Limit Distractions: Create a coding environment that is free from distractions. This might mean putting your phone on 'Do Not Disturb,' using noise-canceling headphones, or setting up a dedicated workspace.
- Time-Blocking: Designate specific periods for focused coding. Use techniques like the Pomodoro Technique to set short bursts of intense work followed by short breaks.
- Mindful Coding: Practice mindfulness while coding. Be aware of each line you write, each problem you solve. This focused attention can often usher you into a state of 'Zen.'
- Structured Breaks: When you take breaks, make them meaningful. A short walk, some light stretching, or even a few minutes of meditation can help maintain a balanced focus.

The Intersection of 'Eat,' 'Pray,' and 'Zen'

Finding your Coding 'Zen' is closely aligned with the principles of "Eat, Pray, Code." When you're in a state of 'Zen,' you are naturally more aligned with your physical needs ('Eat') and mental well-being ('Pray'). Achieving this balance makes it easier to maintain all three aspects in harmony, thereby lowering the risk of burnout.

Conclusion: The Journey to 'Zen' is Continuous

Finding your Coding 'Zen' is not a one-off event but a continuous journey. Just as code is constantly refactored and improved, so too should you continually assess and refine your work practices. In achieving this balanced state, you are setting yourself up not just for short-term gains, but for a fulfilling, long-lasting career in tech that enriches all aspects of your life.

In our final chapter, we will bring together all the components of "Eat, Pray, Code" into an actionable plan for achieving work-life balance in the tech industry. Stay tuned!

Tools and Resources

Apps for Balance

As we wrap up the discussions on 'Eat, Pray, Code,' let's explore some practical tools that can support you in maintaining a work-life balance. In today's digitally-connected world, there's an app for almost everything—including for maintaining a healthy balance between your professional and personal life. Here are some apps that can help you achieve your goals in each of the three pillars: 'Eat,' 'Pray,' and 'Code.'

Apps for 'Eat'

- MyFitnessPal: Track your meals, exercise, and nutrient intake to stay on top of your health.
- Yummly: Find healthy recipes tailored to your taste and dietary preferences.
- Mealime: Simplifies meal planning and grocery shopping with customizable meal plans.
- WaterMinder: Helps you stay hydrated by sending reminders to drink water throughout the day.

Apps for 'Pray'

- Calm: Offers guided meditations, sleep stories, and breathing programs to reduce stress and improve mental well-being.
- Headspace: Provides a wide range of mindfulness practices, including meditations for work, sleep, and stress.

- MyLife Meditation: Formerly known as Stop, Breathe & Think, this app allows you to check in on your emotions and recommends short activities and meditations based on your mood.
- 10% Happier: Features courses and guided meditations on various topics, aimed at making you more resilient, focused, and happier.

Apps for 'Code'

- Todoist: A task management app to help you prioritize and track coding tasks and projects.
- Trello: Excellent for project management and collaboration within coding teams.
- Clockify: Tracks time spent on coding tasks, helping you implement the 80/20 principle more effectively.
- Forest: A productivity app that discourages you from using your phone by growing a virtual forest as you work on tasks.

General Work-Life Balance Apps

RescueTime: Monitors how you spend your time on your devices, providing an overview that can help you manage your work-life balance better.

- Freedom: Blocks distracting apps and websites for designated periods, allowing you to focus better.
- Offtime: Helps you unplug by blocking distracting apps and calls, setting boundaries for work and personal time.
- TimeTree: A shared calendar app to coordinate your work and personal schedules effectively.

Conclusion: Leveraging Technology for Balance

Technology can often be a double-edged sword: while it offers unprecedented opportunities for innovation and efficiency, it can also be a major source of distraction and stress. However, by mindfully choosing and using the right apps, you can turn technology into an ally in your quest for a balanced life in the tech industry.

As you move forward in your journey to 'Eat, Pray, Code,' remember that tools are only effective if used correctly. Integrate these apps into your daily routine, adjust as you go along, and don't forget to reassess periodically.

Thank you for joining us on this journey through "Eat, Pray, Code." Here's to a balanced, fulfilling career and life in the world of tech!

Recommended Reading

In addition to the practical tools and apps that can help you find balance, literature can offer deep insights, strategies, and the emotional sustenance needed for a fulfilling life in tech. Below is a list of recommended reading, organized according to the three pillars of "Eat, Pray, Code."

Books for 'Eat'

- "The Omnivore's Dilemma" by Michael Pollan - An exploration into what we eat and how it impacts us and our environment.
- "Nutrition and Physical Degeneration" by Weston A. Price - A classic book that looks into the diets of indigenous communities and what we can learn from them.
- "Eat to Live" by Dr. Joel Fuhrman - Focuses on nutrient-rich foods and their impact on longevity and disease prevention.
- "Why We Sleep" by Matthew Walker - Not strictly about food, but invaluable for understanding the important role that sleep plays in our overall health.

Books for 'Pray'

- "Wherever You Go, There You Are" by Jon Kabat-Zinn - A guide to mindfulness and meditation, perfect for busy professionals.
- "The Power of Now" by Eckhart Tolle - Discusses the importance of being present and how it can positively affect your emotional well-being.
- "10% Happier" by Dan Harris - A skeptic's guide to meditation and the benefits of a mindful life.

- "Daring Greatly" by Brené Brown - Explores the role of vulnerability in building emotional resilience.

Books for 'Code'

- "Clean Code: A Handbook of Agile Software Craftsmanship" by Robert C. Martin - Offers principles and best practices for writing clean, maintainable code.
- "You Don't Know JS" (Book Series) by Kyle Simpson - A series that goes in-depth into JavaScript, but also teaches broader programming concepts.
- "The Pragmatic Programmer" by Andrew Hunt and David Thomas - Full of practical advice and tips for becoming a better, more efficient programmer.
- "Deep Work" by Cal Newport - Discusses the benefits of deep focus and how to achieve it, particularly relevant for coding tasks.

General Work-Life Balance Books

- "Boundaries" by Dr. Henry Cloud and Dr. John Townsend - A look into setting and respecting boundaries in all areas of life, including work.
- "Essentialism" by Greg McKeown - Focuses on doing less but better, particularly relevant for managing work-life balance.
- "The 4-Hour Workweek" by Timothy Ferriss - While not everyone can achieve a 4-hour workweek, the book has useful advice on productivity and lifestyle design.
- "Atomic Habits" by James Clear - Discusses the power of habit formation and how small changes can make a big difference over time.

Conclusion: Lifelong Learning for Balance

While apps and other digital tools offer practical, everyday support, these books provide the knowledge base you'll need for long-term success and balance in the tech industry. Each recommended read offers something unique to help you maintain equilibrium across the three main pillars: 'Eat,' 'Pray,' and 'Code.'

Remember, achieving a balanced life is an ongoing process, and continual learning is a big part of that journey. These books offer a valuable resource as you strive for a fulfilling, balanced life in the high-pressure, fast-paced world of technology.

Online Communities

While apps and books can offer instrumental support and knowledge, community interaction can provide the emotional and mental backing needed to maintain a balanced life, particularly in a demanding field like tech. Online communities serve as platforms where you can share experiences, seek advice, and provide help to others navigating the same challenges. Here are some online communities that can support you in achieving the triad of balance encapsulated in "Eat, Pray, Code."

Communities for 'Eat'

- Reddit's /r/Nutrition - A bustling forum for all things related to food, diet, and nutrition. Discuss the latest scientific studies, ask for personal advice, or share your own culinary creations.
- MyFitnessPal Community - This extension of the app allows you to interact with other users, participate in challenges, and share tips on achieving your health goals.
- SparkPeople - A comprehensive platform that combines nutrition, exercise, and community support in one place.

Communities for 'Pray'

- Insight Timer Community - Associated with the Insight Timer meditation app, this community offers groups and discussion boards on various meditation and mindfulness topics.
- r/Mindfulness on Reddit - This subreddit offers a space to discuss mindfulness techniques, share resources, and offer support to others trying to cultivate mindfulness in their lives.

- Tiny Buddha Community - This online community focuses on personal development, emotional well-being, and mindfulness, featuring forums and blog posts on various related topics.

Communities for 'Code'

- Stack Overflow - The quintessential platform for programmers, Stack Overflow allows you to ask specific coding questions and get answers from experts in the field.
- GitHub - While primarily a code repository, GitHub also allows for community interaction via issues, discussions, and contributing to open-source projects.
- r/programming on Reddit - A general forum for discussing programming languages, career advice, and coding challenges.
- Dev.to - A friendly and inclusive network for software developers, offering articles, discussions, and collaborative projects.

General Work-Life Balance Communities

- Workplace Stack Exchange - Provides a platform to ask specific questions related to work-life balance, career development, and office etiquette.
- LinkedIn Groups - Many LinkedIn groups focus on work-life balance and mental well-being in the workplace. Examples include 'Work-Life Balance Champions' and 'Wellbeing in the Workplace.'
- The Balance Club - An online community specifically designed for discussing and promoting work-life balance, featuring webinars, articles, and interactive forums.

Conclusion: The Power of Collective Wisdom

Online communities offer the unique advantage of collective wisdom. No matter how tricky a situation you find yourself in, chances are someone else has been there before and can offer some guidance. Furthermore, these platforms give you the chance to contribute your own experiences and expertise, enriching both your life and those of others.

The journey to balance in the world of tech is often fraught with obstacles and stress. But you don't have to walk this path alone. By joining these online communities, you not only equip yourself with additional tools for achieving balance but also gain a support system that understands your unique challenges and aspirations.

So, as we wrap up "Eat, Pray, Code," remember that balance isn't a destination but a continuous journey. And like any journey, it becomes far more enriching and manageable when shared with a community.

Conclusion

Your Personal Blueprint for Balance

As we conclude this journey through "Eat, Pray, Code," it's important to recognize that the quest for balance is not a one-size-fits-all endeavor. Rather, it's an evolving process that will look different for each individual, particularly in an industry as dynamic and demanding as tech. Your blueprint for balance will be a living document, a continuously adaptable guide tailored to your unique needs, priorities, and circumstances.

Reflect, Assess, and Iterate

- Reflect: The first step is awareness. Take time to reflect on your current work-life balance and identify areas where you could improve. Are you eating healthily? Are you dedicating time to mindfulness? Are you managing workloads effectively?
- Assess: After identifying the areas for improvement, evaluate the different tools and strategies discussed in this book. Pick what resonates with you, from brain foods and exercise regimes to mindfulness practices and coding philosophies.
- Iterate: Implement the chosen strategies, but also be open to adjusting and refining them as you go. Balance is an ongoing process, and you'll need to revisit and tweak your blueprint regularly.

Leverage Community and Technology

Don't underestimate the power of community and technology in your journey. As discussed in the previous chapter, online communities can offer emotional support and collective wisdom, while apps and digital platforms can assist in task management, mindfulness, and overall well-being.

Celebrate Small Wins

Balance doesn't have to be a grand, sweeping transformation overnight. Small, incremental changes often make the most lasting impact. Whether it's cooking a nutritious meal, spending five extra minutes meditating, or successfully automating a repetitive coding task, celebrate these small victories. They are the steppingstones to a balanced life.

Be Compassionate to Yourself

Finally, it's crucial to be compassionate to yourself throughout this journey. There will be times when you'll falter when the chaos of life interrupts your plans. That's okay. What's important is how you respond to these challenges. Give yourself the grace to make mistakes, learn from them, and move forward.

The Journey Continues

Thank you for taking this journey through "Eat, Pray, Code." While the book comes to an end, your own personal journey towards balance is just the beginning. Take what you've learned, apply it in a way that makes sense for you, and don't hesitate to adjust as you go along.

Remember, balance isn't a destination but a continuous journey, and you are the cartographer of your own blueprint. Here's to a fulfilling, balanced life in the exciting, ever-changing world of tech!

Appendix

Quick Recipes for Healthy Eating

In line with the 'Eat' pillar of "Eat, Pray, Code," this appendix offers quick, easy, and nutritious recipes designed to fuel your body and mind. Each recipe takes 30 minutes or less to prepare, so they easily fit into a busy tech lifestyle. Let's dive in!

Overnight Oats for a Brainy Breakfast

Ingredients:

1 cup rolled oats

1 cup almond milk (or milk of your choice)

1 tablespoon chia seeds

1 teaspoon cinnamon

1 tablespoon honey or maple syrup

Optional: fresh fruits, nuts, and seeds for topping

Instructions:

Combine the oats, milk, chia seeds, cinnamon, and sweetener in a jar.

Mix well, cover, and refrigerate overnight.

In the morning, stir again and top with fruits, nuts, or seeds before eating.

Quinoa Salad for a Quick Lunch

Ingredients:

1 cup cooked quinoa

1 cup cherry tomatoes, halved

1 cup cucumber, diced

1/2 cup feta cheese, crumbled

1/4 cup olive oil

2 tablespoons lemon juice

Salt and pepper to taste

Instructions:

Combine the cooked quinoa, cherry tomatoes, cucumber, and feta cheese in a bowl.

In a separate small bowl, whisk together the olive oil, lemon juice, salt, and pepper.

Pour the dressing over the salad and toss well to combine.

Stir-Fried Veggies for Dinner

Ingredients:

2 cups mixed vegetables (e.g., bell peppers, carrots, broccoli)

1 tablespoon olive oil

2 cloves garlic, minced

1 tablespoon soy sauce

1 teaspoon ginger, grated

Salt and pepper to taste

Instructions:

Heat olive oil in a pan over medium heat.

Add the garlic and ginger and sauté until fragrant.

Add the mixed vegetables and stir-fry for about 5-7 minutes, or until tender.

Add the soy sauce, salt, and pepper, mixing well.

Simple Fruit Smoothie for Snacks

Ingredients:

1 banana, peeled

1/2 cup mixed berries (frozen or fresh)

1 cup almond milk (or milk of your choice)

1 tablespoon chia seeds

Optional: 1 teaspoon honey or maple syrup for sweetness

Instructions:

Add all the ingredients to a blender.

Blend on high until smooth.

Taste and adjust sweetness, if needed.

These are just a few quick recipes to get you started on your journey to a balanced, nourishing diet that complements the high demands of a tech lifestyle. Feel free to modify these recipes to suit your tastes and needs. Here's to healthy eating and a balanced life!

Coding Hacks for Efficiency

To align with the 'Code' pillar in "Eat, Pray, Code," this appendix provides you with quick, actionable coding hacks designed to boost your efficiency and effectiveness as a developer. Whether you're a seasoned programmer or a newbie, these hacks will help you navigate the often-overwhelming world of coding with less stress and more productivity.

Keyboard Shortcuts

The less time you spend switching between the keyboard and mouse, the more efficiently you can code. Memorizing keyboard shortcuts for your text editor or Integrated Development Environment (IDE) can speed up your coding significantly.

VS Code: Use Ctrl + Space for code completion.

Sublime Text: Use Ctrl + D to select the next occurrence of the selected text.

Eclipse: Use Ctrl + Shift + L to view all the available keyboard shortcuts.

Code Snippets

Reuse common pieces of code by creating code snippets. Most IDEs have an option for storing and easily accessing code snippets.

VS Code: Use the User Snippets under Preferences to create your own.

Sublime Text: Navigate to Tools > Developer > New Snippet to make a new one.

Example: For a JavaScript function, you might have a snippet that automatically generates:

javascriptCopy code

function functionName(parameters) { // code }

Use Version Control

Always use version control systems like Git to keep track of changes in your code. This will not only allow you to revert to previous versions when necessary but also makes collaboration easier.

Basic Git Commands:

git init: Initialize a new repository.

git add .: Add all changes to the staging area.

git commit -m "Message": Commit changes with a message.

Automated Testing

Automated testing can save a lot of time in the long run. Tools like JUnit for Java, pytest for Python, or Jest for JavaScript can help you ensure that your code behaves as expected without manually testing every single function.

Comment and Document

Well-documented code is easier to debug, update, and collaborate on. Though it may seem like it slows you down, it saves time in the long run. Make it a practice to write comments and documentation as you code, not as an afterthought.

Use Task Runners and Automation Tools

Task runners like Grunt, Gulp, or Webpack can automate repetitive tasks like minification, compilation, linting, and more. This enables you to focus more on writing code and less on the chores surrounding it.

Take Breaks

It may sound counterintuitive, but stepping away from your code can actually make you more efficient. Following techniques like the Pomodoro Technique can help you maintain high levels of focus while also giving your brain a chance to relax and reset.

Rubber Duck Debugging

If you're stuck on a problem, try explaining it out loud as if you're talking to a rubber duck (or an actual person). Articulating the problem can often help you see it in a new light and understand it better.

Embracing these coding hacks can make a significant difference in your daily coding activities, making you not just a faster coder, but a smarter one. After all, in coding as in life, it's not just about working hard; it's about working smart.

Contents